Noreen, mother of one teenage son, lives in Cork, Ireland where she grew up as part of a large dairy farming and horse breeding family. She has worked in a variety of educational institutions including her local university as a Director of Studies, Teacher Trainer, and language teacher. She has lived and worked in France, Spain and Mexico during her adventurous career and life path which has led her through other occupations and businesses including high value sales, running pubs plus a restaurant and managing a boarding school. She is currently building her dream as a professional singer and speaker.

This is her first book, a very personal attempt to make sense of a fast-paced, often unbalancing world which can taint us with the sense of never being enough. This learning journey for Noreen is most definitely still a work in progress driven by a knowing that the best is yet to come.

This book is dedicated to my son.

Noreen O Mahony

WHEN SLEEPING
WOMEN AWAKEN

AUSTIN MACAULEY PUBLISHERS™

LONDON · CAMBRIDGE · NEW YORK · SHARJAH

A CIP catalogue record for this title is available from the British Library.

ISBN 9781035801008 (Paperback)
ISBN 9781035801015 (ePub e-book)

www.austinmacauley.com

First Published 2024
Austin Macauley Publishers Ltd®
1 Canada Square
Canary Wharf
London
E14 5AA

When Sleeping Women Awaken, Mountains Move –
Chinese proverb

Dear Reader,

I am so delighted that you are here.

Thank you in advance for considering my words and my message.

My hope is that they will give you food for thought. My words may also act as a useful perspective on how you might be happier on a day-to-day basis and realise that it is your life, no-one else's.

A word of caution though; may I respectfully suggest that you do not believe anything I say.

In fact, I encourage everyone to not believe anything anyone says, be it a single person, an authority or an institution.

I encourage you to consider all sides of an argument, all angles and opinions, and then make your own decisions based on your own instincts and your own innate intelligence.

This is something that we are not encouraged to do by our world.

We are given opinions and facts, and told how to feel and how to react based on other people's claims and opinions.

Most of our thoughts and beliefs come from such a culture.

This means that they do not come from ourselves.

Is this because we believe that we don't know?

Is that true?

Do we not know what is best for our own lives?

These are the questions I'm exploring here in this body of work.

I know that many of the subjects in this book are written about in such a way that may help you to change that way of thinking. However, if something does not ring true for you, it is either because your belief around it is very deep and you are not ready to look at it or because it is something that is not true for you.

All you need to do is to look at whether your old belief serves you by making your life better or not.

By your life I mean your peace of mind, your success levels and your general state as you go about the business of living.

If there are opinions in here that you don't agree with, that is your absolute right.

However, I would ask you to look deeply at those and follow them back to the root.

If they make you uncomfortable, that is a sign that they may be stirring something or awakening old emotions that may be linked to something in your past.

We often think that discomfort is a bad thing but we need to remember that we can only grow outside of our comfort zone. In this circumstance I agree with the adage,

'No pain, no gain.'

However, this saying is often used inappropriately.

It is used to convey the idea that life is a struggle and that everything we do that is worthwhile is painful.

I do not agree with that.

I believe that if we are in flow and alignment, life is easier and more joyful.

It is moving into that state of belief that takes the effort.

If we stay doing and thinking the things that we have always done and thought, nothing changes.

It is sometimes definitely easier to stay in that old familiar place but it often leads to stagnation which leads to death.

By death I mean the death of curiosity, enthusiasm, joy, fun and all the other wonderful parts of life that make it all worthwhile.

I believe that those things are what we came to this human experience for.

Surely we came to grow, expand and thrive!

That is my mission for myself.

By fulfilling this mission, I hope to help others to do the same.

It is not enough for me to talk about doing it, I want to actually categorically do it myself first.

That is why I am writing this; it is part of the process of walking the walk for me, personally.

I know that my work may help not just women but also our wonderful men to wake up to their real power. It is then, and only then, that we can move those mountains.

Of course, maybe your lives are fine, maybe you are happy most of the time, maybe you have enough money, love and success.

If this is you, move on to another book☺

The secret of change is to focus all your energy, not on fighting the old, but on building the new – Socrates

Who Controls our Thoughts?

OK, first things first; it's time to start realising what life really is and how we are creating our own lives by the way we use our thoughts.

It was only in my 50s that I began to realise that most of the thoughts and beliefs in my head were not my own.

They were other people's ideas, beliefs and opinions.

They had been installed in my mind like computer programmes.

This had been happening since I was born and possibly even in utero when I was absorbing the thoughts and emotions of my mother, and what was going on in her environment at that time.

My father was also part of her environment as was my paternal grandmother, so all of these people affected me energetically from the very start of my life experience.

The exciting news that I have learnt in the last couple of years is that I can change these thoughts and programmes if they are not doing me good. I hasten to add that the people in my environment were doing the best that they knew how to do at that time.

If I make these changes, I can change my life to be more of what I want rather than what I don't want.

How exciting is that?

I actually did not know this possibility existed even though I had done a lot of reading and studying in the world of self-development.

When this realisation dawned on me, I was filled with excitement and a new zest for life in my 50s.

I realised that part of my life's work, maybe all of it, is to share this message with the world.

For me it is easy to do this through speaking, writing and singing.

This aforementioned "dawning on me" took time, effort, financial investment and faith.

It did not happen simply or just by reading about techniques in self-help books, doing meditation, journaling etc. (though these now form part of my daily life), I needed hand holding to get into the deep stuff.

My coaches, mentors, healers, advisors and teachers all played a major part in this journey and my heart is filled with gratitude for each and every one of them.

You know who you are!

It often makes me smile when I think of how easily we spend money on clothes, hair, holidays and so on yet baulk at investing money in getting to know our deeper selves.

We make excuses, we say things like "I don't really believe in all that", "I don't have time" and the list goes on.

My hope is that you will do some of this work.

What happens, as if by magic, is that when you make the decision to do it, the right teachers/mentors/guides will show up at the right time.

The huge mistake that people make is that they wait for the favourable circumstances before making the decision.

They have it the wrong way around.

Make the decision first, this is vital.

When you make the decision, it is only then that the universe can start to work with you.

Read this again as it is so important.

What is needed then is the courage and faith to take that step.

I am always delighted to help people to make a start on this journey of wisdom and compassion into themselves.

If a coach/mentor does not suit you, you will feel it and following your own intuition is a fantastic way to start this process.

Building trust in ourselves is key to expanding our consciousness.

If you don't feel the connection to your mentor, find someone else or what usually happens is that the perfect teacher comes into your life effortlessly.

But remember this can only happen if you have already made the decision to do the work.

What is consciousness you may ask?

It's a good question and one that is difficult to define.

For me, at this moment in time, consciousness means my thoughts, feelings and actions.

I now know that fear contracts it and love expands it.

Let's look at it in relation to modern times.

It is the year 2021 and we have just finished a most extraordinary period of time across the world.

There have been huge changes for a lot of us in the way we live our everyday lives.

Many of us feel that we are not in control of our lives right now.

Many of us believe that our governments, our health authorities or other people are in control.

The good news is that only you can control your own life and you can start this very minute.

In this book, you may get some glimpses into the secrets of how to achieve peace in your head, a more abundant outlook on life and a new appreciation of who you really are.

These times are a wonderful training ground for teaching your mind not to react to the outside world but to go within and listen to your soul.

We have been brought to where we are now for a reason, everything is as it should be.

No matter how difficult that may be to believe, I urge you to consider it and see if it makes you feel better or worse.

That is how you know if something is serving you or not.

You do not need to believe me or anyone else, consider all viewpoints, then go within, research and make your decision based on how it makes you feel.

It is important to remember that you may be addicted to bad news, this is very possible.

You are in the habit of listening to it and it has become so familiar that you are unconscious of your relationship with it.

You are not alone.

Millions of people across the world are in the same boat.

However, you can alight from that boat any time you like.

The choice is yours.

It is the mark of an educated mind to be able to entertain a thought without accepting it – Aristotle

How do we Begin the Change Process?

First of all, we have to take responsibility for our own lives. We have been trained to believe that outside forces are responsible for our lives, our health, our finances, our wellbeing, our children's education, our family background, the economy and the list goes on.

This is a mindset, the aforementioned programme that has been installed on our minds.

It's like a set up.

We have been coerced into thinking like that and it is often painful to realise and accept this.

So it's time to be big girls and boys and start taking life by the scruff of the neck and saying to it, "actually, I'm in charge here".

I will do my own thinking around this, my own research and then decide what to do. I will also tune into my Creator and see what S/He has to say about it.

I will get advice from people who may have more experience than me but ultimately, it is my decision about how to proceed.

Can you feel the energy of these statements?

Do they make you feel empowered or weak and out of control?

You know by the gut feeling which answer is right for you. You may not be ready to embrace those feelings right this minute but the fact that you entertain and consider them is a start.

Well done you!

Sometimes saying them in a nice gentle way is not enough. We might have to shout at our thoughts or even scream at them to get out of the way.

Something that helped me was to say, 'There's a new bee in town.' Haha, it really helped me to get rid of the old thoughts.

The earlier in the day you can start doing this the better.

For example, when we open our eyes in the morning is a good time.

What is the first thing you think about?

Are you going to have a good day?

This is a decision that you can make at that waking moment. The alternative is to look at your phone and see the news, social media etc. telling you about the problems that are in the world.

If this is what you do, then you are setting your vibration for the day.

You are also setting the vibration of your environment and everyone around you.

The knock-on effect is that your day gets off to a negative start.

You allow what is going on externally to determine your internal world which, like a domino effect, infects your thoughts, words and actions which ultimately cause your results. This is the basic message of Bob Proctor and many more.

This leads us into the world of our vibration and different frequencies.

From the above example I'm sure you can understand whether you are in a high or low vibration, if you start your day with negative thoughts.

Negativity vibrates at a low frequency.

If you are vibrating down there, you attract in people, circumstances and events of a similar low frequency.

It is therefore vital to keep your vibration as high as you can for as much of your life as you can.

How do we do that I hear you ask?

By doing things that make us feel good, by being around people who bring up our vibration and by being people who bring up other people's vibration.

A saying comes to mind: *If you bring the light to others, you cannot keep it from yourself.*

Of course, being up there 100% of the time is probably not possible nor desirable for most of us.

It is the flow of life, with all its ups and downs, that makes it interesting and helps us to keep growing and expanding.

I'm sure you can remember feeling these vibrations before. Think about a day when something very special was happening, a birthday, a wedding, a special occasion etc., you wake up with a feeling of good excitement which can feel like nervousness as well.

That day starts very differently than the day you look out of the window at the rain and decide "it's miserable"!!!

Think about what we are saying to our deeper mind when we say things like that in our heads, and worse again out loud.

We are inviting in a "miserable day".

I usually say, "it's a great day for the ducks or the grass".

I try not to allow the weather to determine my mood, I am the master of my own destiny.

Florence Scovel Shinn tells us: *Your word is your wand*, so we need to be very careful how we use them.

They in turn affect our vibration and can take our frequency up or down.

If we stay focused on this fact during the early part of the day, this is where we can really make a difference.

Moving on to the bathroom in the morning.

You look at yourself in the mirror.

What do you say?

'You look great,' 'I love you,' – probably not!!!

It's more likely to be, 'You look awful,' 'Your hair is a mess,' 'You are fat,' and the list goes on.

You do not say these things out loud, they are secret thoughts that you tell nobody about.

You probably are not even aware of them most of the time. This is the voice I have already mentioned.

It has to be stopped!

You would never ever admit having these thoughts to your friends and family, hardly even to yourself.

However, if you even start to become aware of them, you are on the road to recovery on so many levels.

Can you change these thoughts? Oh, yes, you can!

You can start by copying me.

I say, 'Today is going to be a lovely day with lovely surprises,' 'I love you Noreen,' 'I love your body because you are strong and you carry me every day where I want to go.'

'I love you belly because you provide the space for all my digestion to happen which feeds my physical being.'

Furthermore, 'You carried my son for 42 weeks and kept him safe.'

'I love you breasts because you make me feminine and curvy. I love you extra fat because you protect me but now I am happy to let you go because I know that I am always safe, and I do not need you any longer.'

'Thank you for all you have done for me.'

This is part of my story.

You know your own story or at least you are starting to investigate it, so you start to tell yourself that new story.

Imagine how different your day will be if you adopt a few of these practices in the morning.

Imagine yourself coming to the kitchen in that vibration to have your breakfast.

Do you think the day will go well?

It has a much higher chance if you take the time to direct it in the way you want, rather than letting it to chance, external circumstances or other people.

Of course, there are always days that do not go well but tomorrow is always a new day and we get the chance to start again with a fresh page.

That's what sleep is for.

It is like a washing machine.

It washes out the stains and dirt of yesterday.

A Chinese proverb says: *The longest journey starts with the smallest step.*

These are a few steps that I am giving you as examples because they have helped me.

However, we have to be brave enough to take that step.

If we choose (and it is always a choice) not to, we stay in the same place.

We can think about taking the step, talk about taking the step, dream about taking the step, plan to take the step but if we don't actually do it, the journey never starts.

What is so exciting about this work is that it doesn't matter if it's the wrong step.

The next step can be adjusted, tweaked or corrected to go in the right direction.

That's what courage is, taking that step.

I have taken many steps in my life and had to correct them. My life is all the richer for the steps that needed correction more so than the ones that were perfectly placed.

Do you know… that the "only" thing that makes life hard is… "our thinking" – Fiona Downes, Mindset & Manifestation Coach

Why do we Believe Others' Negative Opinions?

One of the most damaging and contaminating phenomena in our lives can be other people's negative opinions. I learned this from the great Napoleon Hill.

By people I mean those around us, the media, the government and anyone who gives us information in any form.

The funny thing is that often when people around us compliment us, we often don't believe them.

These compliments are positive opinions.

They tell us we are looking well, doing great things or that they are happy to see us and we don't take the time to acknowledge these positive comments.

We often do not believe their opinions in those instances but we have no problem believing the negative ones.

Why is that?

There are many reasons from a myriad of psychological studies, theories and scientific facts.

These vary from an addiction to negativity possibly, deep programming of the mind which has been passed down through our DNA and reinforced between the ages of 0 and 7 years old by our primary carers and the environment in which we live.

That is a whole other area of study which I would encourage you to investigate if you are interested.

In this book I am focusing on raising our awareness around these topics and shining the light on them, so we may better see them in ourselves by doing our own investigation.

Referring back to other's negative opinions:

How many love stories were never begun?

How many inventions never happened?

How much money was never invested?

How many jobs were never applied for?

How many boys or girls never dated?

How many people denied themselves the pleasure of each other's bodies because of guilt, fear and shame?

How much energy was wasted on listening to people who really did not know what they were talking about?

They were, in fact, only expressing their own fears and limitations based on their own life experiences.

How many times did we settle for second best because of what someone said?

How many exciting risks were never taken out of fear of being criticised by others?

I'm sure you can add to this list from your own life.

What is the way forward?

It can be done gently but firmly.

You might practise by saying; "this is what I'm doing and while I respect your opinion, I'm going to do it anyway".

"If it is not the right step, I'll correct it but at least I will have no regrets or resentment towards anybody for stopping me".

This method I have used myself with some success.

The first time is difficult but then you get used to doing it and people around you get used to your new way of being.

Often people stop us because they have their own view of the world and they want us to have the same one.

Often they think that they are trying to protect us from failure, disappointment or even disgrace.

They do not realise that they are asking us not to be selfish but to do what they want us to do!!!

Funny isn't it?

So when we ask for others' opinions, we are actually asking for permission, approval, validation or a mix of all three.

We do not trust ourselves.

We need approval from a family member, partner or friend.

Studies show that 80% of our actions are done for approval. I would contend that it is higher than that for women.

Sometimes we are the wo/man who stops ourselves and this goes back to our own negative beliefs as discussed in an earlier chapter.

It is that little voice in the head telling us the same old stories.

If we make changes in our lives doing this kind of new work, people will notice and some negativity may flow towards you from some quarters.

This is because your self-improvement may be acting as a reflection of other people's own feelings of inadequacy or weaknesses which they are afraid to tackle or even acknowledge in themselves.

You are upsetting the status quo.

Throughout history we know what happens to people who do that!

They have been villified, ridiculed or worse.

Watch out for it and don't be surprised if it is very close to home.

Send out the light of compassion to those who may be blinded by your increased brilliance.

You may help them to adjust their settings to see the brilliance in themselves.

It is so important to remember that you will never do it if you don't shine yourself.

The journey between who you once were and who you are now becoming, is where the dance of life really takes place.
– Native American Wisdom

Are we Human Doings or Human Beings?

I've just finished reading some of Neale Donald Walshe's wonderful book "Conversations with God" and I got a fresh angle on why Covid has been such a gift for so many of us.

It forced us to stop doing, doing, doing.

There has been a huge release and relief for a lot of people because the pressure is off.

Possibly this has been more of an issue for women than men. In my experience I see women struggling more with that.

Women's sense of value in themselves seems to force them to try to do it all.

Our self-worth is tied up in the doing.

Here is the list that many women follow:

The job, the children, the slim body, the perfectly applied make up, the exciting social life, the good wife, the good housekeeper, the good cook, the soft skin, the large circle of friends which means you're popular, the landscaped garden etc.

Within each of these items is another list of doingness e.g., children need to be protected, educated, skilled up in sports and music to within an inch of their lives because their competence is a direct reflection of mother's worth.

Whew!!! Isn't it exhausting?

Now what's interesting in this are the stories we tell ourselves about it being good for the children.

If we really stop and analyse it, we do it to make ourselves feel better by keeping up with the neighbours, friends etc.

Of course, children need a certain amount but not to the extent that mother is exhausted by it all.

So what has Covid done for us?

It has helped us to "be" more than to "do".

Our mornings are slower, we take time to enjoy breakfast.

The house does not need to be so tidy or clean because nobody is coming around to visit so no one will see and I will not be judged. Here I am speaking personally and I know that not everyone feels like that about a clean tidy house.

I don't need to put on make-up or uncomfortable clothes or shoes because I have nowhere to be.

If I do have an occasion to get dressed up, I enjoy it more knowing that I can relax again tomorrow into not doing much.

I am looking in the mirror and getting used to seeing the real me without all the trappings.

I actually have time to look in the mirror!

I am learning to smile at myself and say that all is well in my world.

This is a deep knowing in my soul because if I were to listen to the world around me, I should be stressed and fearful listening to ever-increasing numbers of disease and contamination.

However, I know my own truth. I am slowly realising that my thoughts are what dictate my life.

I choose peace.

While all of that sounds lovely and fluffy, how do we put it into practice?

In the world of this moment, the vibration is definitely low for many more people.

I am embracing the opportunities to help people to lift themselves.

How am I doing that?

By staying as high as I can myself and spreading my vibration as I walk, interact and be.

I choose to move around as freely as I want to.

It is so interesting to me how people really believe that they "cannot" travel and that they have to follow guidelines that are not serving them.

This is a similar belief to the Irish girls who went into mother and baby homes, and believed that they could not leave or do it any other way. This did not just happen in Ireland of course but has been highlighted more here possibly.

Their mothers and fathers had the same beliefs.

These beliefs came from society and the church, which was the local government of the day.

These were seen as the people in authority and their rules were followed unquestioningly by society.

The same thing is happening now.

If you point this out to people, they can get angry.

They have accepted this belief and there is no changing it.

"It is true, it is reality" is what people say in defence.

My reality is different because I am making it so.

Grant it, it is more challenging in these times but I am having some success.

I know that I am a healthy adult with a strong immune system and I pose a threat to no one.

People who would judge me as selfish are living much closer to fear than I am and that is their choice.

We can live in whatever emotion we want.

That is the beauty of free will.

It does not serve me to live like that so I choose not to.

Of course, it has taken me time, and the help of many great women and men to learn that but girl is it worth it!!!

I know that by living like that I am happier, healthier and I can be of more service to my fellow woman or man.

I get feedback on that every day.

I try to help people to rise – the song "Rise Up" by Andra Day springs to mind.

I'm going to listen to it right now before I go on.

Have a listen and see what you think!

One of the best ways to raise that vibe is through feelings of gratitude.

This has been scientifically proven and can be researched online.

This is part of my day now.

I do not necessarily sit and write it, though I know this is very important and so I try to do it more and more.

I try to have it as part of my thought process and it is now becoming more automatic.

I can now enjoy the fabulous house that I have without complaining about its faults.

I am using and enjoying the state-of-the-art kitchen that our mothers would have dreamed of while they were cooking and feeding 4/5/6+ children, plus husbands.

I appreciate the comforts that I have around me more and more and realize that I do not always have to be acquiring or buying things in order to feel happy.

However, I can spend money on improving my home too because I realise that my environment can be important to my feelings of well-being, "being" being the operative word. It is finding the balance and it is a thin line I know.

I am learning how to be well while "being" rather than "doing".

This is an enormous realisation for many of us and it is a lesson that will hugely benefit us if we foster the practices.

Another area where I feel grateful is around friendship.

In my opinion during pre-Covid times many of us did not value the importance of authentic human connection and interaction. We wasted our time on false relationships perhaps while not nurturing the important ones.

What are the important ones?

The ones that make us feel good.

That is how we know.

Easy isn't it?

You know those people that when you walk away from them, you have a sweet taste in your mouth, a lovely feeling inside. Those are the ones worth valuing.

In the past we were possibly running so fast trying to get everything done, we may have missed that nugget of wisdom and awareness.

As the song says we need to slow down as we were moving too fast.

Thank you Covid, whatever you are!

Life seems a quick succession of busy nothings –
Jane Austen

Was Lockdown the Key to Freedom?

It's Sunday morning and I feel totally free to do what I really want to do today.

I can light the fire and watch movies, I can cook, I can visit family, I can go for a drive, it is a wonderful feeling to have the freedom to do what makes me feel good today.

This is a luxury that we can enjoy, thanks to lockdown.

The shops are closed, work is closed, people are not expecting us to be here, there and everywhere.

People are staying home mostly.

For many people this is a relief from the stress of their former lives where they were constantly under pressure. Many people have said to me, "2020 was one of the best years I've ever had".

However, people feel guilty about saying it because the story we are being told is that it's very bad, we need to feel scared, we are in danger etc.

The reality is that many people realise this is not the case but they feel that they have to go along with that story even though it may not be true for them.

Yes, there are some people that are getting sick as they do every year and some people die, as they do every year.

The difference is that now we are being given these numbers on a daily basis by the media.

Remember, we always have a choice to listen or not.

If it makes you feel bad to listen, maybe try not listening. This is a habit we may find difficult to break but give it a try and see what happens.

During 2020 many of us realised that the way our lives were moving was not really in the direction that we wanted.

What is interesting about this is that most of us career through life without ever really asking ourselves the question, "what do I really want"?

But when lockdowns were forced on us across the world, everything stopped.

We could not continue the running and racing, filling our lives with often meaningless activity.

We now have a chance to reset.

It is up to us whether we embrace the opportunity or not.

People hopefully have a new appreciation of the value of socialising and how important it is for us.

People now appreciate the pubs/bars and catering industry in general more and the role they play in our social lives.

I believe that as we re-emerge, we will be happy to pay more for our quality food and appreciate the labour, time and money that goes into handing us even a simple cup of coffee. I see that happening already.

A coffee has now become a treat for us and we savour it all the more.

This is good.

Going to our local bar or restaurant was something we took for granted, maybe we complained about the prices or the variety on the menu.

Now we will be delighted to go back there, happy to see the owner and happy to pay for the service we get.

We now value the service that is provided for us, not just in the consumption but in the social interaction it affords us.

My hope is that there will be a whole new energy around "going out".

People have had to spend much more time in their homes than ever before.

This has been very beneficial for a lot of us.

Many of us have invested money in our homes and in our gardens to make them nicer for ourselves and our families.

This brings us pleasure.

We know that this is not the case for everybody, and we know that for some families it is not easy but I think that because there is nowhere to run, families are learning to reconnect with each other in a deeper way.

On the other hand, some relationships are not going to survive this test.

If that is so, end it as cleanly and compassionately as possible for all parties involved and start afresh.

There is no point in flogging the proverbial deceased equine!

There is definitely much more home cooking happening and this by its nature is bringing people closer.

It's happening in my house with my 13-year-old, we are being forced to connect with each other and it is good for both of us.

It is not sunshine and roses for everyone and we always have to acknowledge that. Living in rural areas or smaller countries has been much easier than in big urban areas of course.

However, feeling guilty about our own happiness does not help anyone, least of all ourselves.

If we can raise our vibration, it helps everyone around us, neighbours and the wider world included, to feel better.

This is quantum science and there are studies which prove it if you care to investigate and research.

If everyone is thinking alike, then somebody isn't thinking –
General George Patton

Is Marriage a Myth?

If we look at the origins of marriage, it is difficult to get real clarity because of course, the reasons for marriage have changed over the years.

It used to be based on ownership, possession and property. It was also used to unite families to give them more status, security and wealth.

What's interesting is that the whole "love" idea is very recent as many of you probably know.

I used to think for a long time that marriage was made for men and by men in a time of totalitarian patriarchy. I am not so sure about that anymore and something is definitely changing.

We all know only too well that marriage was at times, a fairly toxic environment for many women in the past. What is interesting in modern times is that it may now be quite toxic for a lot of men also but this is not something we discuss as women and I think men discuss it even less.

I find it fascinating to wonder why we continue with ideas and "traditions" with a "one size fits all" approach when it clearly does not.

For example, many of the ceremonial symbols and practices reflect another world than the one we live in today.

Why do we want to continue with them?

Why do many women continue to take on their husband's name (even as double barrelled)?

Why do we wear rings to symbolise the fact that we are owned?

Perhaps you see it differently or maybe you've never thought about it at all.

Why is the bride often handed over from father to husband?

The white dress, let's not even go there!

If it doesn't mean anything really, then why don't we change it?

Why do we still pass on this archaic model of the world to our children, in particular, our daughters?

Symbolism is very powerful and it programmes our sub-conscious mind.

The big industries and religions know this and use it to manipulate and/or control us.

But we also use it on ourselves, often without knowing.

This is very true around marriage in my opinion.

At least the men sometimes joke about it, calling their wives the "ball and chain" or joking about running away before the big day.

The women do not generally do this.

Why not?

It's all very serious stuff.

She loves him.

Everyone around her approves of this.

It's the thing to do.

It gives respectability.

It's important for children.

It doesn't matter if the marriage is dead in the water, you stick with it as long as possible.

Thankfully in the western world, these ideas are becoming less prevalent but many of the old ways and beliefs still exist in the symbolism as well as in our own minds.

I think it's a great idea to examine all these beliefs, unpack and sort them, and keep what serves us.

In my own case, I have never married but I have really wanted to up to very recently.

Since I have really looked hard at why I might want to have had that label of being "married"; I realise that it was just that I'd have liked to fit in with that club for a while, to be a member.

I used to believe that I would like the formality of it, the public commitment of my love so that the outside world would know.

The secret thought is that he would be mine, he can't go off with anyone else (haha, we all know where that can lead), he helps me to pay the bills, buy/rent the house, raise the children etc….

So much of it is still about property and ownership if we look at it closely!

Our culture still tells us(women) from birth that we should aim for marriage.

It is talked about with little girls routinely whereas not much at all with boys in my experience.

Why is that?

Is it seen as more important for women because they need to be minded/protected on some level in order to give birth and take care of baby?

Of course women need support around children, from pregnancy to child rearing but nowadays, they often do not get this support from partners who have to work or extended family who may not live near.

Again this is an area that is not really discussed with young women or men.

It just happens by accident and they are left to navigate the complexities of it by trial and error.

There is no practical guidance at all for couples or single parents.

Getting back to the marriage question, in my opinion, it is often the women who want to own and control in the modern marriage, at least in western society where that is possible for them.

Many men seem to have lost their power, and the whole system has wrestled it off them and handed it to the women which perpetuates the whole control and ownership illusion.

We see this very clearly in marriage breakdowns and child custody battles.

The legal system fattens, the couple stew in hostility and hurt, and many children look on in bewilderment and pain.

This is often compounded by one or another parent speaking negatively, even poisonously about the other parent.

This can cause untold damage on a spiritual and psychological level in the child.

We hear how damaging divorce/separation is for children. This is only true if we make it so.

We can tell a different story to our children if, and only if, we wake up and get honest with ourselves.

Women do not need men to protect them in the modern world but it sure does make life a lot easier if we have a supportive partner around to share the load.

Men should not be judged as more stable by being married or that they cannot take care of their own needs without a woman.

However, raising children is definitely easier if there are two people working as a team.

I have no doubt about that and I'm sure you have all seen examples of that in your own life experiences.

In my own case the teamwork came from my family members rather than a partner, and because of that support, it was an easier road for me than for other single parent families…

I was mature enough to ask for the help, and that was a great advantage of being older and wiser when I started the motherhood journey.

I believe people should only get married and stay married if they are helping each other to grow.

If that stops, if one is stopping the growth of the other, it's time to move on.

Wow, imagine how freeing that would be!!!

Imagine the absence of heartache and hurt if there was no judgement or commentary by society.

Furthermore, the children would know no differently.

The wow exclamations would be if your parents still lived together by the time you were 15.

If they did, you knew it was because they really wanted to, liked each other etc., it had nothing to do with you.

Whew!!!

No pressure.

The reality is that couples are applauded for longevity in a marriage even if one or both are just joylessly existing, going through the motions, waiting for retirement into old age and death; is that what life is really supposed to be all about?

We deserve to have so much more but we do need to start taking those all-important steps towards it.

Don't get me wrong, I think a good marriage is a wonderful thing for both parties.

I also believe that life is easier if it is shared.

We know this from any experiences where teamwork is involved.

It adds fun, connection and productivity to the game.

The idea of marriage is a good one in that two heads and two pairs of hands are better than one.

But those heads and hands have to be working in unison.

In Celtic times I have heard that the marriage contract was 9 years. After that you could choose to renew or not. (I cannot find this information on a simple online search but this is not unusual. The information published is often what the powers of the day want or don't want us to know).

What freedom!!! Do you agree?

Should marriage be for life?

Everything changes, so do we right?.

We have to in order to stay growing but often between couples, one stifles the other.

As Mr Wilde said: *Yet each man kills the thing he loves*.

Of course there are bumps along the road and running for the hills as soon as that happens is not the answer either.

We need to attempt to move through our lives with joy and fun as consistently as we can.

That's my recipe though I do not always succeed.

Will you allow yourself to make it yours too??

I hope so!

How can we even begin to start that courageous journey? Well, we need to go deep within and really feel curious about what we believe and if those thoughts serve us or not.

It is not for the faint hearted hence the adjective "courageous".

An interesting conversation I had the other day with a friend on the subject was; what if both parties are happy to go along in mediocrity?

I suppose that's fine, is ignorance bliss?

I'll leave that for yourselves to consider and decide.

Have that conversation the next time you're out with the girls.

You might be surprised by what comes up.

I would be delighted to be a catalyst for these conversations particularly as I am more in the dark on this subject than many of you readers.

Many of our men would also be interested in having these discussions if we can hold a safe space for them to do so without judgement.

Our modern world encourages war between the sexes in subtle ways that many of us are not aware of.

We must reunite the Divine Feminine and the Divine Masculine in order to evolve more I believe.

I invite you to consider these points and when you do, you will know instinctively if it is close to your own truth or not. If it isn't, discard and move on to other considerations but never stop considering.

That is the way to your own personal unique truth.

"Romantic" love is not enough in the union of two people, you need respect and a curiosity about yourself and your partner. You must be willing to grow together – Author NOM

What is a Woman's Sexual Organ?

After the topic of marriage, let's get down to the red-hot topic of sex!!!

Before starting to write this, I thought I had better do some extra research on women's sexuality because I realised that I did not know very much about it.

Isn't that strange? I am a 55-year-old woman who has had a child but I felt I didn't know enough about my own sexuality. What I learnt from a few super Ted Talks by learned women absolutely amazed me.

The following videos on YouTube were fascinating;

Cliteracy by Sophia Wallace
The Unknown Greatness of the Clitoris by Maria Rosok
The Pleasure Principle by Laurie Betito

I found out that the female sex organ is the clitoris.

I half knew this but not really if you know what I mean. No-one at home or at school had ever actually taught this information.

I don't believe it is being taught as part of our children's sexual education today.

I find that quite extraordinary! How much and yet how little has changed around this life area.

Since this revelation I have been asking everyone I meet if they know the answer to this chapter's question and 1 out of 15 get it right!!!

Can you believe that?

We do not know what the female sex organ is.

I have got answers like the vagina, the breasts and the brain.

Other fascinating information is that the clitoris has almost as much erectile tissue as the penis.

75% of it is internal and the full mapping of this organ was only done in 2009.

While the penis has 300,000 nerve endings approximately, the clitoris has 800,000.

I was flabbergasted by all this information that I did not know.

I had struggled with my body image, weight and feelings of low self-esteem most of my life like many people.

I would even say that most women feel this way for the first half of their lives, many until their deathbeds.

Some do come out of it in middle age and my work will hopefully help more to awaken to their sexual power and pleasure.

It's never too late!

I then began to realise that a lot of these feelings can be traced back to the stories we were told and our interpretation of what our sexuality is as women.

This came from our parents, probably our mother first, followed by father and then society as a whole.

We were only told about the dangers of sex (pregnancy, reputation, STIs etc.) and we were never spoken to by anyone about the pleasure that our God-given bodies can give us.

Any exploration of this is shrouded in shame, comedy and vulgarity.

This is also true for men but at least their sex drive is acknowledged and we know all about their organ!!!

In the past and well into the present as I have found out, the woman's organ was thought to be the vagina whose purpose was to receive the penis.

This does not lead to much pleasure for women as there are very few nerve endings in the vagina and contrary to what you see in the movies, it is not a case of sticking it in and she writhes in pleasure.

Now I understand why so many women felt that there was something wrong with them sexually because they couldn't achieve an orgasm with penetration alone.

The fact is only 20% can do that so 80% of us may have been missing out on the pleasure which our bodies are designed to give us by not being well acquainted with our clitoris and its importance.

Needless to say, many men have no idea either and that has led to much lack, frustration and loneliness in this department of relationships.

I remember being instructed as a child to feel shame about my genitals.

"Shame, shame" was actually said if I pulled up my dresses or showed myself in any way, while out running around the farmyard free as a bird, as more children were in those days.

This was at the tender age of 3 or 4-years-old.

This was before I had any sexual thoughts, urges or knowledge.

The other day I had a great conversation with a friend of mine who has always been super open about her own sex life.

I was telling her about this chapter and she was surprised to think that she was an exception when it came to discussing her own female sexuality.

She has always known to take control of her own pleasure by using an extra object to get to the important places.

It was so refreshing to speak openly about it all while taking it seriously and having some fun at the same time.

You know how women can do that!

Let's get this conversation going women and men!

It does not have to be a fight, it is not about wresting power from anyone, there is plenty of spiritual and sexual power to go around.

Our sexuality is possibly the most powerful part of who we are and this is the same for both sexes.

We have been given the wrong information for centuries.

It's time to change this very important story.

Let's get this party started, one clit at a time – LL

Who Told us we are
not Beautiful?

We have been told for years, decades and even centuries that we are not enough as we are. This is more true for women than for men I think.

We have been told that we are unclean because we menstruate.

We have been told that our bodies are imperfect, too tall, too small, too skinny, too fat, too angular, too soft etc.

We have been told that we need any number of potions and lotions to look and feel our best.

We have believed it all.

The vast majority of these aforementioned potions and lotions are very lightly regulated with regards to toxins and other harmful substances which we liberally apply to our skin on a daily basis.

In the last few years I have become more and more aware of the issue of health around skincare and the beauty industry.

The use of deodorants with metal has been highlighted but many of us continue to use them because they are handy and easy to use.

We cannot allow any of our bodily natural smells to exist! We think they are disgusting, that means we are telling our body that we think it is disgusting.

What I have found is that since I have stopped using anything under my arms, the smells have virtually disappeared.

If I have something particular on which may cause extra perspiration, I use a natural product to get me through the day.

Nowadays I am not obsessed with showering every day, If I am staying at home writing for example, I allow my body and skin peace.

If there is any odour, I give thanks for my body's ability to excrete any waste substances or toxins.

That is what our glands and skin pores are for.

If we block them or put extra toxins on them, the body cannot do its job efficiently and there will be consequences.

I do believe that this is a big problem as well around our hair dyes and hair products.

Do some research for yourself.

I have brought all my products to my stove side chair of an evening and studied them with a magnifying glass as it is often impossible to read the ingredients.

I do this for my health and well-being and it is much more educational than Netflix!!

My perfume these days are essential oils like lavender.

I wash with natural soaps free of the nasties.

I walk about in my natural fabulous odour which is unique to me.

As women we often compliment each other. Sadly our men are probably afraid to say anything complimentary to women nowadays in case of misinterpretation.

'Your hair is lovely,' 'Your dress is gorgeous,' 'You've lost weight,' 'You look great,' these compliments come out of our mouths so frequently that we don't give them a second thought.

Let's look at these compliments in more detail.

Are we taking our value from how we look or what we wear? Many of us are and it is not our fault, we have been told that this is the way we should be.

Our sense of self has been conditioned and programmed into our sub-conscious minds by corporations including the beauty industry, the entertainment world and the food industry.

This self-image then determines the thoughts we hold about ourselves.

They have been recorded in our deeper minds and we believe them to be true.

This manipulation has been happening for decades, particularly through TV and magazines, films and music. These industries are powerful and nowadays particularly, in the hands of a few corporations. I have recently been watching movies from the 1930's and 40's and I see it more clearly.

This goes back to an earlier chapter about our self-talk – what we say to ourselves in the mirror (we don't necessarily need the mirror, any self-reflecting surface will do, a window or other shiny surface).

We don't even need any reflection because we have ingrained it on our minds so it's always there.

Can you change it?

Oh, yes, you can.

How do we do that I hear you ask.

We do it by realising that we are not our hair, or our bodies or our face etc.

We live in those things; they are simply the packaging and trappings that we need to navigate this human life.

We are much, much more than that.

We are divine beings of consciousness living within this vehicle called a body.

Of course, we need to take care of it and it is important in so far as we want it to last as long and as healthily as possible so that we can better experience everything that life has to offer.

In other instances many of us reject these compliments when they come.

We shrug them off or say something self-deprecating.

Why do we do this?

Why can we not accept the compliments?

Is it because we don't really believe them, because we don't want to seem boastful or arrogant or because we don't feel it within ourselves, so perhaps we feel like a fraudster if we do accept them?

I have at last realised that I am not my body, which incidentally has carried too much weight for decades.

I now know that I am a spiritual being on this most marvelous of journeys and I am releasing everything that was weighing me down, including the weight. This is a process and I still have a way to go.

Am I the same wonderful being, perfect in my imperfect expression of life that I have always been?

Yes, of course, I am.

Do the people who loved me love me more now because of my lighter, stronger healthier body?

No, absolutely not.

Those who really love me see the same energy, spirit and fun that was always there.

So what has changed?

I have changed my self-image and I'm still working on this.

I stopped seeing myself as the "heavy" Noreen, that little girl who had always been told she was big.

How am I doing that?

By working with amazing coaches who help me to open up to my higher feminine self which is ultimately connected to God /Creator/Universe.

And girls, is this a fun place to be!!!

Deep down I always knew S/He was there as do you, I'm sure but I had to make the decision to rediscover and allow that reemergence.

I would not be writing this book if that hadn't happened, no question about it.

I had done every diet in every book.

One time I dropped 7.25 stone (46 kilos/101lbs) in 16 weeks.

It was a total food replacement programme, not the healthiest thing to do for lots of reasons but it allowed me to see my bones and the actual structure of my skeleton which I had forgotten!!!

I went on to pile all the weight and more back on again because, of course, in my subconscious mind I was still "heavy" Noreen.

No amount of dieting, starvation or food regimes could fight against that picture in my mind.

Since the self-image has improved, the weight has started to release as I build a new image of a new woman.

I've had to change the way I lived and ate and drank.

If we want to become someone different, e.g., a light, fit, strong Noreen, we have to change our habits and this can be scary.

Is it doable?

Oh, yes, it is if you really, really want it!!!

In the past I had tried to start with the body in order to make the mind feel better but I was doing it backwards. Now that I know better, I'm doing better.

I started by working with an amazing personal trainer who saw me as the athlete I really am, and who told me that I was dead and disconnected from the neck down.

How right he was!!!

He said this with compassion because he knew that I was ready to hear the lesson.

We work in the gym to bring light back into and through my body and more importantly to stop the mind.

My muscles needed to wake up.

My weight loss is not yet where I want it to be but I know I have to persist because the alternative is unacceptable to me.

I try to be gentle with myself and I allow the process to run its course. At the same time I know that it is what's in my subconscious mind that will get me the results I want. It is also connecting with God/Creator/Source and that's the only effort I need to make.

The difference this time is that I do not go into the old narrative of beating myself up as I had done down through the years when the scales failed to move, or only moved up and down or up, up, up!!!

Over the past decade or so I have done a lot of research into the food industry and I am convinced that it holds the key to our physical health.

I now try to eat food which is not processed. By processed I mean, unchanged by human interference.

I endeavour to eat organic as much as possible but I know that the label organic is not always what we think.

One does have to be brave to ask the growers of our food what exactly they use to enhance growth or appearance.

What I find interesting in this age of information is how hard it is to find out what is added, sprayed or injected into foods which we assume are unaltered.

My inflammation is now reducing (often weight is a sign of inflammation).

The wonderful thing about being overweight is that it is an outward symptom of internal inflammation.

Slim people may also suffer from inflammation but it is not so obvious, so I am grateful to my body for showing me the signs so that I can correct and heal as much as possible.

As I take all of these different steps, the path unfolds ahead of me and I find other great teachers who help me to continue this journey of self-re-education.

It wasn't really "discovering" because the woman I am has been there all along, I had just become disconnected from her.

I would like to remind you at this point of the importance of taking those steps, we cannot advance without doing the study and learning to unlearn.

One of the universal laws of the universe is "action" and it is often not highlighted enough in my opinion.

Without action, nothing can change.

Now some of you may ask me why I can't love myself as I am. The answer is I do love myself exactly as I am today.

However, that love started before any weight releasing happened.

It has to. I had been trying to do it the wrong way round all my adult life. Now I do love myself regardless of how I look or feel. However, I want to feel and look fully alive.

I want to live the rest of this life being the best I can and having the most fun I can.

This can only be done if I am in the best physical health possible, and this is a choice that we all have. I know it is not easy and it seems that the odds are stacked against us but we have to dig deep within and find that super God-given power.

I hope my story inspires you to do the same.

Let food be thy medicine, thy medicine shall be thy food – Hippocrates

Whose Health is it?

"Your health is your wealth" is a phrase that trips off people's tongues very easily but methinks that we know very little about what health really means.

Our beauty is intrinsically magnified by how healthy we are and how healthy we feel.

One does not need to be a nutritionist to know that what we put into our bodies is going to have a huge impact on our health and longevity.

There is the idea that because we are living longer, we are healthier.

That is not always true in my opinion.

Many of our older people are medicated very heavily, shuffling around crippled with arthritis and going from doctor's appointment to doctor's appointment only to end up in a nursing home, sitting on a chair waiting for life to end.

Is this living longer and better?

I think it's a question we need to ask ourselves.

In the nursing homes (by the way there is one nurse per 30 patients in Ireland so even the name is misleading) neither the patients nor their families really know what they are being prescribed.

In many cases it's sedatives and other medication which deadens, not only their bodies but also their minds and spirits.

This is not necessarily the fault of the homes, though we know some have been found guilty of neglect.

We again have handed over the responsibility of our older folk to the state so it is we who are setting up these systems. The food in these homes is generally processed with little or no fresh fruit or vegetables.

This is the same in our hospitals as any of you who have spent time there can confirm.

This is certainly the case in Ireland, it may be better in your part of the world and of course, institutions vary hugely depending on who is leading the team.

Serving sausages and bacon (known carcinogens) to physically vulnerable people is really not for their good, and again we say nothing.

We remain asleep.

The information on the dangers of certain foods is now available if we take the time to look for it. I know there is confusion but we do really need to clear up this confusion by doing our own research.

We are in the age of information, let's take advantage of it.

It becomes the norm to accept low standards and we don't even question it. However, deep down we know it is not right.

Families cannot agree with each other and so Mum or Dad has to go into care.

They then explain to you with big eyes that there was no other way.

These comments will no doubt anger some of you who have been in this situation but this is not my intention.

I also know that in some cases an institution like a nursing home is the best solution for your loved one particularly near end of life.

My intention is to jolt you into thinking outside the box – excuse the pun!!!

I thought it was so sad that during 2020 our old people were prisoners in institutions that their families could not access for months on end.

I know that if I had had anyone in such a place, I would have broken them out regardless of the consequences.

It has made me realise that nobody belong to me will be allowed in the doors of these places.

There are undoubtedly people who have no choice because of family relationships or lack of them, but I think we need to make provision for people who will care for us at the end of our days and not leave our possessions divided equally among our children in order to avoid conflict.

Leave them to the person or people who will act in our best interest.

This needs to be done by women especially, as we outlive the men statistically speaking.

Ladies, keep control of your assets and think long and hard about who will care for you.

It would be easy for someone to give up a job if they stood to inherit a house for example.

If the government then exempted such people from inheritance tax, the situation would be quite different I believe.

As an aside, I have recently realised that the governments' game is money so there probably won't be tax relief in that area.

There is always another way of looking at situations and the belief that we cannot look after our older people in their homes or our homes is not serving them when they are at their most vulnerable.

Equipment can be brought in, extra help can be contracted if preparations have been made in advance.

Exhaust all options before handing them over.

Have the courage to have those conversations, woman to woman.

Ireland is a country that has an appalling track record of caring for people most in need in our society. We seem to have short memories about many of these scandals.

Other areas of health where I regularly raise my eyebrows is when I hear conversations among people in their 50's/60's/70's about this operation, and that ailment, this medication and that immunisation programme; which the manufacturers admit may have long term future side effects. Many of these dangers are not explained and we are told that we have no way of knowing future consequences.

Again this information is in the small print which is given to us by the pharmacists but it's as if we do not want to know about them.

We just believe what we are told.

It's like people are sleepwalking and sleep talking without really thinking about what they are doing or considering that there may be another approach.

If everyone is having the same problems, then what is going on?

It seems standard practice now to be put on blood pressure and/or cholesterol tablets as early as your 50's.

Why?

Is there not a natural dietary solution?

Of course there is but we have handed the control of our health totally over to the medical industry which is governed and funded by the pharmaceutical industry.

It's like a badge of honour to be listing what meds you are taking.

We think that there is no other way.

We do not dare question the medical profession.

It's a bit like the infallibility of the church in the past.

All the while we can access the real information online that many of the tests and studies are outdated and downright incorrect scientifically or have been funded by the very businesses that manufacture them causing serious conflict of interest.

Cancer comes under this category as well.

People believe the narrative that it is incurable or can only be treated with the mainstream drugs.

The truth is that we have the cures for many diseases but they are being silenced, censored or discredited. Again the approach is a "one for all" when there is a mountain of evidence to show that this is not effective. Do your own research and see what interesting information you find.

Once a cancer diagnosis is made, the patient is thrown into a whirlwind of procedures and treatments without any real discussion or alternative perspectives.

There is no discussion about diet, alcohol consumption or what may have caused these dysfunctional cells to thrive in the first place.

The wheels of big pharma are put into motion and God nor woman will not stop them, or so we think.

If a person dares to question or ask for time to consider, they are frowned upon and one feels the raised eyebrow-disapproval of the mighty medics.

Again I am not saying that these medical treatments do not have their place but there are always other options to be explored.

Take the time to do your research, ask other people's opinions who have been through the same or similar experiences.

Most importantly, listen to your own intuition by getting beyond the fear that such a diagnosis can cause to rise up within us.

Our doctors do not know everything, they are trained in institutions which have been funded by huge corporations whose aim is profit, so that is all they know in many cases. Find out how much nutritional training your doctor got for example. How much do medical students learn about food and its impact on our health in today's colleges and universities around the world? It might surprise us.

This is not about attacking our doctors, who are doing the best they can, but about taking back control of our own health.

Our lives begin to end the day we become silent about things that matter – Martin Luther King Jr.

Are we Really what we Eat?

Don't worry!!!

I'm not going to advise you to go out and plant your own vegetables in the garden but I am asking you to consider what we are actually feeding our bodies.

If you search for the top 10 carcinogenic foods, you will see the good old Irish/English breakfast in there.

Yet we continue to feed ourselves and our children sausages, bacon and other processed meats.

Are we just ignoring the scientific facts?

I drive a diesel car.

I know that if I put petrol into the tank, it is going to cause my engine serious problems.

That is what most of us are doing every day, several times a day.

We are putting diesel into a petrol body or vice versa.

So let's look at it.

Nowadays when I go into any supermarket, I look up and down the aisles and realise that most of what is on the shelves is not real food at all.

We have been led to believe that it is by a powerful industry which has infiltrated the highest levels of politics and health systems globally.

What most of the products contain are quantities of sugar, bad fats and chemicals that over-stimulate our taste buds, cause cravings due to their addictive properties and inflame our bodies on multiple levels.

Most of us do not take the time to research any of this information, it is available if you dig deeper than skin level, and follow the trails.

I would strongly encourage you to do this for the sake of your future health.

It is literally a matter of life and death.

It is more a question of a life half lived in sluggishness and brain fog; and a prolonged, often painful end of life.

Unfortunately, as already stated earlier, our doctors get little or no training on nutrition during their studies and this is causing untold suffering for millions of people across the globe.

In my opinion, these Covid times have given us many valuable lessons.

We were forced to cook more when many of us might have been eating take-away meals, or eating out several times a week.

I know I was not cooking my own food often enough and I am not an exception.

It has been a great reset for me personally and I will not be going back to my old ways.

I also realised how much less food we need if it is real food. A few potatoes: steamed or boiled, some unsprayed vegetables and grass-fed meat is a very healthy meal.

In Ireland we have an abundance of good beef and lamb which has been raised humanely for the most part.

Finding the unsprayed vegetables may prove harder but it is possible.

I have personally changed my shopping habits to make regular trips to my local farmers' markets and farm shops.

I find that I value the food more, I waste less and savour it while I'm eating.

If it costs a little more, I am happy to invest that in myself.

Overall, I find myself saving money as I am not buying the other stuff in the big shops.

We must go back to eating food in its most natural state.

Sometimes I think people don't understand that unprocessed food is food unchanged by human hand.

Now there is the whole question of GMO foods but I'm not going into that here.

It is a subject for a more scientific writer.

There is a wealth of information online and in books, start educating yourself, listening to your body by noticing your energy levels and start to make small positive changes to bring you back to your full magnificence.

To remember who you are, you need to forget who they told you to be – Native American Saying

What is the Real Deal with Alcohol that we Refuse to See?

One of the problems that these times have caused is that people are drinking more alcohol in the home and for some families, this is an area of difficulty, even crisis.

In Ireland, like in many parts of the world, many of us have a bipolar relationship with alcohol if we are honest with ourselves.

We love it and hate it at the same time.

We love it while we are drinking it but the day after is the problem.

The hangover from hell!!!

What does alcohol do to our vibration?

It brings us down in the long run.

It's confusing though because in the short term, while we are drinking, it gives us the false sense that we are raising our vibration and having fun.

The more we drink, the lower that vibration and sense of fun becomes eventually.

It is a false high – we know that but it is considered to be the only way to have fun for many people in many parts of the world.

This is a belief that we have and I personally held the same thought for many years.

It is the same story with any beliefs that we hold, if they serve us, that's great.

If they don't, we can change them.

Changing our behaviour around alcohol is challenging. People expect you to drink, people put pressure on you to drink and if you refuse; you are seen as "no fun, boring etc.". This is the reality for many people, especially the younger among us.

Our governments and mass media promote alcohol all the time because there is so much revenue in it.

If the goal was to promote health, they could not nor should not do that.

It has been scientifically proven that alcohol causes cancer among other serious diseases but we never hear about that from the medical world (unless you are a chronic alcoholic).

I was so surprised and shocked to only recently realise that alcohol is a group 1 carcinogen.

I believe it is something we should look at in ourselves.

Is the enjoyment worth the aftermath?

Can we consume alcohol without abusing it? For me personally this is difficult. I am an all or nothing woman. Of course I know that it's not all my fault as alcohol is an addictive substance so it's designed to make us want more.

Deep down do we feel we have a problem with controlling it?

We can change our alcohol story if we really want to.

The first step is always awareness.

If we want to make changes, all the resources are there.

Talk to someone you trust or say nothing to anyone and find online support.

We all know what the best path is for ourselves so it's about trusting your own deeper instincts.

Do what works for you.

I wrote the above before reading "The Naked Mind" by Annie Grace.

Wow!!! What a study on the reality of alcohol!!!

All the science is there, all the cultural insights are there and she says it straight, alcohol is poison.

How many of us squirm in our seats on hearing that?

How many of us say, "I drink in moderation"?

So that's the same as taking small amounts of arsenic "in moderation". Think about it!

A number of years ago I read Alan Carr's book on alcohol and he educated me at that time.

The problem is that it is so much part of our culture, that it is challenging to cut it out.

It is the most dangerous drug known to man and yet we have to justify to others why we do not drink it.

Isn't that interesting?

In my own life now I rarely drink it but from time to time I slip back into the old patterns and the little voice in my head says, "go on, you can treat yourself".

I now know that I do not need it to have fun but it is a process that I continue to work on.

During these changing times, I want to have a clear head every minute of every day.

However, if I do have a drink, I do not beat myself up like I did before.

I gently say to myself, you will know better next time.

Like many Irish people there has been alcoholism in my family but what many of us will not admit is that it is still there, no matter how we try to glamourise or normalise it.

For women's bodies the science shows that it is more dangerous in that our bodies get damaged faster than the mens'.

We ignore that advice at our own peril.

Shoulders back women, we do not need the booze to feel fabulous.

Approximately 3 deaths per day in Ireland are alcohol related. (HRB.ie)
In the US 2015-2019, 380 deaths per day were alcohol related. (CDC.gov)

What can I do with the Down Day?

Just in case you think that all my days are high vibe days, don't worry they're not.

This is a good chapter to follow on from the alcohol one as in the past I used to use alcohol to help me feel better.

Now I try to do differently.

Today was a wet cold Irish day and when there is nowhere to go and no one around, it is challenging to stay upbeat. What I have learnt is to not fight that feeling.

If you get into a downward mood, just go with it and do what you feel like doing.

Watch movies, eat what you want and always remember tomorrow is a new day.

I am not advocating not seeking help if you need it, of course. Here I am talking about those days when you cannot seem to get out of your own way.

The energy is low and you feel like doing nothing.

Going out for a walk is too much effort, cooking something healthy would feel like too much of a struggle, ringing a friend for a chat?

Can't be bothered!!!

On those days I feel that if I ring someone, I will bring them down so I prefer not to.

Abraham Hicks says: *It is generally better to not fight that momentum and to wait for a new day.*

When I heard that it gave me a sense of relief.

I now feel that I can just take it easy and go slow, live those days on my terms so to speak.

I don't have the energy to pretend to be in good form.

Blah!!!

So what do I do now?

I meditate, it may, but not always, pull me up.

I listen to hypnosis or music, that often helps.

I push myself to go out, even very briefly, that can feel better while I am out but can then change down again when I come in the door.

I chat to some neighbours, momentary relief.

I watch a TV series, mind numbing which can also work for a time.

Now I'm writing about it which gives some ease as well but I think the best thing for it is to go to bed early, read a bit maybe as my brain is fried from the TV and go to sleep.

Tomorrow is definitely a new day and I will do everything in my power to start it in a cleaner vibration.

What's interesting is that sometimes, none of it works and now I am able to accept that.

Before falling asleep I set the intention to wake up in a better mood.

The moment I wake, I am determined to start the day differently.

Then I proceed into the shower to wash all the old energy down the drain.

I put on some nice organic face and body cream, fix my hair and put on a bright top.

I do all this in a gentle way rather than with my usual dogged cross-with-myself approach.

I treat myself like I would a beloved child.

I am more serene and say to myself, "this will shift at the right time", which it eventually does.

I now understand that I have the power to turn it around and I am able to do it faster and faster. As I edit this I have also learned that if I connect in with God, it is easier still.

Now it takes a day or two to shift, before it might have been a week.

Soon it will be an hour or two maximum.

Every day in every way I'm getting better and better. This is an affirmation I use which often helps me.

You can control any situation if you first control yourself
*— **Florence Scovel Shinn** (The Game of Life and How to Play it)*

Why am I Studying a PhD in Me?

The great illusion of education really amazes me.

I have been thinking about this in the context of me, and I realise that I have done a PhD in me over the last 4 years in particular.

What does that mean?

It means that I have really intensively studied myself, my own behaviour, my reactions to what is happening around me, how my childhood affected me, how I thought about myself and so much more.

Through all of this study and application of practices which focused me on my inner world, I am beginning to see the illusory nature of what I used to think was a real world.

I now see that life is a set of systems set up by a few unseen people who may not always have our best interests at heart.

However, because of the work that I have done and continue to do on myself, I now see it much more clearly.

Another gift of Covid is that for many people this fact has come out of the shadows and become visible, for many of us, perhaps for the first time.

Again thank you, Covid.

I now believe in my own standing as a woman on this earth and I now more fully understand what that means.

I have a divine right to be on this earth, to be free and abundant and in control of my own destiny which is ultimately in the hands of God.

That gives me a huge sense of peace in my soul and fire in my belly.

I now live life with more of a sense of trust, a sense of unhurried pleasure that makes every day a little sweeter.

Of course, there are days and moments when that is not the case, but I now have tools to help me regulate during those times.

I am human after all but I have learned and am learning every day to raise my consciousness and keep my heart open.

That is the way to ensure the systems around me fail to control me.

I want to be of service and if that means working as a carer for older people, driving children to school or doing a coaching session with someone; it is all the same really.

One job is not more important than the other.

I do it all while being fully present and serving whoever I am with to the very best of my ability.

I am not superior or inferior to any single living woman or man on this earth.

If I wanted to go back into the education system to get an actual PhD in psychology, for example, I would be lectured by people who have probably not done the work or research into themselves that I have done.

I am not saying that there would be nothing more to learn but I would carefully assess my teachers and not rely on letters after their names on their office doors.

So many of the women around me think they need to do more courses and get more qualifications to do business or give advice to others when they are already experts in certain fields.

The authority that teachers/lecturers have is many times well placed but just as often misplaced, and I think we need to remember that.

Like I have already said, we should not believe what people say but consider it, question it and reject it or accept it based on our own perspectives and intuition.

In my opinion, our youth are encouraged less and less to think for themselves.

Much of the learning is propaganda, and has an agenda to keep them dumbed down and obedient in order to become good employees within the system.

These are strong words but if we scratch under the surface, we may find truth in them.

This is particularly true in the areas of science, medicine and education itself.

There is a great Ted Talk called "Do Schools Kill Creativity" by Sir Ken Robinson, and other videos and articles about how our school systems are built on the Prussian model.

Have a look at those and see what you think.

During my own time in the education system, both as a student and a teacher, I enjoyed it.

In school as a student, I was interested in languages and literature, and so the system suited me as there was no great difficulty in those areas for me personally.

I did not, however, learn how to manage my life in any meaningful way.

I was not taught financial literacy, how banks work or how the taxation system works.

I was not encouraged to be a businesswoman, but luckily I come from a business-minded family so that knowledge was there to some extent.

Nothing much has changed in this regard in modern times.

As a teacher I was trained in how we learn, and I was fascinated by how my international students thought, what they thought, why they were sitting in front of me and if they were happy or not.

I wanted to know about their opinions of Ireland and the West.

I encouraged them to think critically, to consider different perspectives, not just in class but in all aspects of their lives.

In school I did not learn about my own personality, my own family background influence on my view of the world or anything that would help me to make life as great as possible.

All this study started after I left university.

Are our young people today ready for this information?

Yes, they are in my opinion but our teachers are not equipped to teach them and the system does not want that knowledge imparted.

You might want to ask yourself why that is.

We need a new system or maybe no system.

As parents we need to realise that we are our children's best teachers and education is not about memorising information that is not always true. For example, history is written by the victors and edited by those who own the media. These corporations may be following an agenda.

What is this agenda?

May I suggest that you do some research.

Start by looking at the topics in your children's schoolbooks.

What are the messages that our children are absorbing?

Some of this information may not be immediately obvious if you do not know how the mind works.

The first step for parents is to learn about themselves, what makes them tick, what gives them joy, what is killing them physically, mentally and spiritually.

As I review that last sentence I wonder if "killing" is too strong, maybe "dumbing down" is better.

I'll give you the choice!!!

This work is not for the faint-hearted as I have already said.

However, we owe it to the next generations so that they can reclaim their power and rightful place on this earth and live a less burdened existence.

For my yoke is easy, and my burden is light – Matthew 11:30

What is your Role as a Parent?

Is parenting the most selfish or selfless endeavour?

We parents often think that we are amazing.

We think that we are so self-sacrificing and noble.

Why do we have children?

To have someone to love us?

So that we have someone to love?

Or to own?

Or to control?

Or to force to do the things that we couldn't?

Or to educate to within an inch of their lives?

Or to show off to our friends and family?

Or to be admired for and clapped on the back?

Or to be part of that great eye-rolling club on the street or in the supermarket when children don't do what we want them to do?

Here I am borrowing some of Doctor Shefali Tsabary's ideas which really made me think about this and consider what she says.

I do not agree or believe everything but there are very interesting perspectives which have helped me to relax about my own parenting, especially around the teenage years.

I realised that I didn't want my child to miss school because it would make me look bad as a parent, and I was afraid of judgement from his teachers and other people around me.

I knew in my soul that he was fine and not missing anything major that would positively impact his life going forward.

I really knew in my heart and soul that school was doing more harm than good in the area of creativity, self-expression and self-esteem.

This has been made even more clear to me, and I know this is the case also for many parents, in recent Covid times.

So let's really look at the "system" that is in place for the majority of families in the Western "civilized" world.

We put our children into childcare as young as 4 to 6 months.

In Ireland there have been scandals about the treatment of children in such institutions (yes, they are institutions parents!!!), it was news for a couple of days and then people went merrily about their business again.

It's good for their development you will hear parents say and their socialisation.

I am sorry to say but all experts who are honest say that a child needs their parents as their first teachers.

Deep down we know this.

My heart breaks for the mother pulling her child out of bed at 6:30am to be put into a cold car and dropped to the childminder or creche.

I don't care how nice they all seem to be, your child is not winning, you are not winning and ultimately the universe is not winning.

We have no idea what the long-term effects will be on society but like everything else we don't like to look at, investigate or use our critical thinking skills on; we will refuse to link it back.

We will pass the blame on to technology, the modern world (which we have created by the way) and anything else we can think of.

Remember, you don't have to accept my opinions, just consider what I'm saying.

Life is not black and white, there's lots of grey in there.

From the childminders/creches they go to playschool at age 3 or 4 where they line up, follow the rules and listen to authority figures.

Then it's primary school, uniforms, books, crayons etc. I remember my sadness as I left him there, in the hands of people who I knew very little about, whose ideology was probably totally different from my own with the little tie wrapped around his little neck.

Instinctively I knew it was not for his good but if you said that to anyone, you would be ridiculed.

I believe that's why many mothers and some dads cry at the school gates on that first morning, deep, deep down they know.

They smile sympathetically at each other, feeling each other's pain.

By the rest of society they are often dismissed as over sensitive, I said it to myself.

I now apologise to that God-given intuition which was possibly trying to tell me that I was on the wrong path.

I kept my tears until I sat into the car but I didn't know what they were for.

Often us mothers dismiss ourselves because we cannot articulate what we really feel, even to ourselves.

For centuries we have been told that being emotional is weak, that it makes us women weaker than our male counterparts but we know differently and so do our men. They know it makes us strong, loving and powerful on so many levels.

During these early years in the state school systems, learning issues may be highlighted and labels put on.

The boys often find it hard to sit still and this causes problems for parents.

They may feel shame that their child is not conforming. What happens to the boy?

He loses the joy of learning because they are all expected to learn the same way.

I noticed this in particular in mixed sex schools.

It has been proven that the system favours girls whose reading and writing skills develop at an earlier age than their male classmates.

There is apparently an enzyme that doesn't kick in in children until age seven which is connected to writing in particular. This is particularly true for boys as far as I know.

A book that I used to research is "Proust and the Squid" by Maryanne Wolf.

I would highly recommend doing your own research even though this information is not so easy to find.

I was lucky to have had really great teachers with my son, and I did the research so he was never told that he was slow or less intelligent because of his delayed writing prowess.

I know that other children are not so lucky, and the fun and enjoyment is gone out of learning well before they reach the age of 10 for many of them.

A belief has been installed that they are not "intelligent" and so the next decade of school becomes an endurance test.

How sad is that?

Are we seeing the consequences?

I believe we are; in the rise in anxiety, depression and suicide in our gorgeous boys and men.

Fortunately, this does not affect the boys in the jobs market, as they still do better than the girls from the point of view of salary and promotion.

So when we hear how important education is, don't always believe it.

Moving on to after-school activities, many modern parents in the western world believe that their children need to be doing 4 or 5 extra-curricular activities per week.

I got sucked into this myself but I always limited it to 2 per term.

I used to see him after school, lying on the sofa and really resting after all the activity from 8am (the time he got up) until 3pm (the time he got home).

I imagined the children who stayed on after school until 5 or 6pm when parents collected them, and wondered when these children had the chance to rest.

Many of them would have been out again an hour later for music or sport.

Now I can feel the anger rising in you reader!

I can hear you saying, 'How dare she!!!'

'What are we supposed to do?'

Well, you are supposed to stop and really look at why you are doing it this way.

Is it just because everyone else is doing it?

Is it because you don't want to lose your career?

Is raising children not a career choice?

Why not?

Why did you have children?

Go back up to the questions at the beginning of this chapter. Let me hasten to add that I am not standing in judgement of anyone here with anything I say.

Are our children becoming more or less confident?

Is their mental health improving or going backwards?

How are their social skills?

I know from my own personal experience that many of our teenagers in particular are really struggling.

Are we brave enough to really look deeply within ourselves to find the answers?

If we don't, we are doing our children a huge disservice.

My wish is that I help my child to successfully navigate our changing world and have every opportunity possible to do that.

I believe that that is the wish of most parents.

I believe that 2020 has given us a new perspective.

I think many of us have seen what is taught in our schools and the wool has been lifted from our eyes.

The system is doing the best it can, but we are not taking responsibility for the children we have brought into the world.

In Ireland, like many other countries, we know what the state can do to the most vulnerable in society.

We have the proof and we are doing it all over again.

This will be discussed in the future by our children and our children's children, and they will wonder at our ignorance or denial, or both.

This year I have offered my 14-year-old boy the option of home schooling.

I really do not want him staying in a broken and worse, tyrannical system.

However, he does not share my point of view and wants to continue in the system for now.

He pointed out the hilarity of the role reversal with him begging to stay in school and me saying not to bother!!!

As I dropped him back for his first day, I watched all the masked children in dismay and prayed that they would not be too harmed in body or mind.

I was in high stress all that day.

He was of course contaminated by my stress so when he came home, very little was said.

I wanted to vent, shout about how crazy it was, but I knew I would be hurting him even more.

I suggested we go to the gym instead where I could squeeze the anger out through my muscles.

It has crossed my mind that people who do not have children for whatever reason, are the advanced beings among us.

They do not need to be needed.

They do not need smallies to feel whole.

Now I know that some people who cannot have children feel deeply disappointed and often sad.

I would ask them to change their perspective if they can and see it as some kind of special recognition from the universe that they are the chosen ones!!!

In my own case, I have one child which might mean that that was enough for me to learn the lessons.

I was one of eight myself so that may be another reason lol!!!

I would not have had the courage to write about these observations if it weren't for Doctor Shefali Tsabary, so thank you Doctor for taking this topic out of the dark so that we may examine it.

I understand that many may not be ready for this but my work is to speak about what I see before my eyes, and what I know from some research and my own personal experience.

You do not have to agree on any level but I hope it helps you to relax a little around child rearing...

It may lead you out of the systems and into a new freedom.

A word to the thousands of teachers out there.

So many of you are doing wonderful work with our young people.

The system is rigid and becoming increasingly so as most of you know.

You are the ones who can start the change from the inside out.

This is not an easy task as you are controlled by the powers and it depends on the culture of your particular school which is often set by the principal/head teachers.

Remember your classroom is your world and you are the guiding light there.

Continue to shine your light and make a difference.

Your students will often only remember how you make them feel about themselves, as Maya Angelou often said:

This is much more important than any other information that you teach.

Thank you from all the parents who forget to say it.

Education is not the learning of facts, but the training of the mind to think – Albert Einstein

Why do we Fear Birth?

It makes me sad that so many women, babies and fathers are deprived of the spiritual experience of what birth is.

It is nowadays cloaked in fear and stress, at least in the developed world and almost fully medicalised.

Much of the problem is because of the horror stories some of us women recount because of our traumatic experiences. Some of the fear comes from tales of the old days that we have heard or read about.

Some comes from the silence, the stories that are not told by mothers who feel some sort of shame around their birthing experience perhaps because it didn't go smoothly, like in the movies!

These stories or non-stories then educate the next generation of women into a mindset of fear and trepidation which in turn leaves them feeling powerless.

They then feel that they must do as the doctor/nurse/midwife says or as their mothers say. Nowadays however, mothers of birthing women are nowhere near their daughters.

Women are very seldomly encouraged to go within, do their own research and decide how they want to experience birth. Many of these decisions are not even mentioned, it's like you are blindfolded and led to whatever the medical world decides is right for you, your body and your baby.

Much more research often goes into planning a wedding, buying a house or even a car than planning the birth of your child.

I went through this process myself at the ripe old age of 40! I educated myself beforehand, I got advice from friends who were willing to talk about their positive experiences but those women were few and far between.

I realised that the majority of women have negative and often traumatic birthing experiences.

I am lucky to count as a friend a professional community midwife and her support was invaluable.

It was the main reason that I had a most empowering, joyous birthing experience, one that I will never forget.

I love talking about it – in appropriate circles – and telling my story to women and men who will listen, and hopefully use it to empower themselves and/or their daughters, sisters, granddaughters etc.

A friend who had had two natural births in hospital after being induced was my guide and doula.

I wanted someone with me who had had a wonderful experience rather than someone who might be in fear because of past trauma, lack of knowledge or lack of belief in the female ability to birth.

This was the most sensible and logical course of action for me at that time and it is one of the greatest choices I have made in my life.

Thank you, Maeve.

I went to the hospital prenatal course which was mediocre in that it went through the logistics and facts but practically nothing on the emotional side of what was to come.

I had the wisdom of my midwife friend who suggested investing in a private tutor who took me for 2 full days of training on breathing, focusing etc. in order to have as natural a birth as possible.

That was what made all the difference.

My community midwives also coached me on being open to all eventualities, including hospitalisation if necessary.

This subsequently happened as I went two weeks overdue.

I accepted this without question as I was informed that one moves into a different risk category.

I am not saying that medical intervention is not needed, of course it is in certain cases but this should be in the minority of cases surely.

Instead women are made to believe that their bodies are not capable of doing this most wonderful of work, unaided by chemical intervention.

This belief is being passed down from generation to generation and so the cycle continues.

This brings me to another issue which may be controversial! In my opinion modern women in the modern hospital birthing process lack the support of another woman-relative or friend while giving birth.

In the old days, this was seen as women's work and the men were excluded.

There was a certain wisdom in this and a lot of relief for the men possibly!!!

However, we can and should have both; our partners and a trusted friend or doula.

What is the big issue with having them with us at the most important times of our lives.?

Nothing of course, but women are not educated in the wonderful benefits of having both types of support and are afraid or not confident enough to state their wishes once they get into the medical realms.

Only we women can change this by making our voices heard.

In 2005 I had a miscarriage at 9 weeks.

I was 39 years old so I was at the stage when I knew that having a baby might not be part of my destiny.

I accepted this and when I miscarried, I said to the universe, OK, if this is the path, so be it.

Five months later, when my relationship was coming to an end, I conceived.

It may have been the last time I was with my partner and bingo, baby on board!!!

By seven or eight weeks into the pregnancy, I was going it alone (relationship finished) and that didn't bother me too much, though I was sad and hurt.

The baby was the light at the end of the tunnel.

At 30 weeks approximately I realised that I would be able to have a home birth.

I had previously thought that because of my age, weight etc. that I would not be allowed.

Even the fact of needing permission for our choice of birth is crazy if you really think about it.

My midwife friend soon put me straight, there would be no problem at all.

My pregnancy was smooth right up to 42 weeks when I knew that I would have to go to the hospital for induction.

I had accepted that this might happen so there was no issue. I went in, was induced, told them no epidural as I did not want my precious baby being pulled out by the head (apologies for being graphic but it is a reality).

The statistics told me that there is a seventy per cent higher chance of intervention with epidural.

I had also done the study of how the body provides its own pain relief if not interfered with, and off we went.

Baby came out with some work (that's why it's called labour) and I felt amazing, like a superwoman.

He was home for his 24-hour birthday because I had everything set up at home, and I told the lovely staff that I was leaving.

They did look at me differently and with some amusement as they were not used to women stating what they were doing.

It was more usual for women to ask for permission!

My declarations were not done with any arrogance, I had great fun with the staff and other mums.

I now realise that because I had taken the time to study and prepare, my confidence was unshakeable.

Often we do not think for ourselves; we allow others to do it and tell us how things are.

This has been very evident in recent times.

We are our own best doctors, midwives and health professionals but we have forgotten it.

So women and men, remember childbirth is a natural process that our bodies are designed to do perfectly.

Trust yourselves and make your own decisions like I did.

If intervention is needed, allow it but make sure you have done your homework so you are fully empowered to make those decisions from your own instinct rather than from a place of fear.

We need to tell a different story around birth. We are going backwards in this area I believe but it is only us women who can change that.

There is power that comes to women when they give birth. They don't ask for it, it simply invades them. Accumulates like clouds on the horizon and passes through, carrying the child with it – Penny Armstrong & Sheryl Feldman, A Wise Birth, Pinter & Martin (2007)

Have we Forgotten what Death is?

During 2020 we heard a lot about death and dying, which in my opinion was really hyped up by our mass media across the world.

My silent questions when hearing this narrative were like, 'Don't we all have to die sometime?', 'Nobody can live forever right?', 'When we reach 89 or 90-years-old, surely we know that we are nearing the end?'

For some people, the end comes much earlier than that I know but hasn't that always been the way of life and the world?

People die every day everywhere.

It is, of course, sad when we lose a loved one at any stage, but when they have lived a long life, do we not need to accept it? Can we describe it as a "tragedy"?

Our modern take on death is quite interesting and I think that we really need to look at our attitudes around it.

No matter how educated or worldly we are, most of us still fear it, refuse to talk about it in any profound way and look to external sources to prevent it or make it less "messy".

We also believe that we can control it.

Yesterday I was reading "Conversations with God" by Neale Donald Walsh and he reminded me that it is the soul that decides when it's leaving.

What does this mean?

Can we alter it?

Maybe we can but perhaps only for the right reasons.

Not if we are afraid, not if we don't want to leave our loved ones, but possibly yes, if we want to expand and thrive more.

This is the jurisdiction of God in my opinion but again, if we let go of the fear, there will be much more ease and flow involved in that final transition.

A friend who has been through the cancer journey commented to me the other day that she hates people saying that someone "lost the cancer battle" because it is seen as some kind of failure.

This goes back to what I just wrote.

Death is not failure.

Have we forgotten?

Death is a natural part of the human experience.

It is actually success.

We came, we saw, we remembered who we really are. Unfortunately for most of us this does not happen until the very end.

We don't remember until we are at the exit, or as Abraham Hicks often says, when we croak.

She has helped me to realise that I want to know this knowing before I get to the "croaking" stage.

I'm having fun and joy now, and enjoying all life has to offer as much as I can.

Referring back to the death stage, let's look at its medical care and end of life care.

Our palliative care systems in the developed world have many wonderful aspects and the majority of the care givers do great work.

However, sometimes I feel that the process is interfered with too much.

Fewer and fewer people die at home surrounded by their familiar environments and people.

It's like we cannot bear to look on as someone takes that final journey.

Many people at the end of life are thrust into unfamiliar surroundings and tended to by strange faces at a most vulnerable time in their human journey.

There is often a lot of stress and fear, because the families and loved ones are afraid to keep control in the medical worlds.

We tend to hand over our control to these environments as I have said in earlier chapters.

Death has become a medical process rather than a spiritual rite of passage just like birth.

Undoubtedly there is a place for medical intervention, but again not always.

I think we are forgetting that.

In 2020 we saw a lot of trauma around this all over the world.

People were forced to die alone and families were forcefully separated.

We need to remember that we are never separated, we are always connected whether we realise it or not.

If we realise it and acknowledge it, the suffering ceases or at least, lessens.

We need to be quiet and tune into that knowing at times when circumstances prevent us from being with loved ones at their time of passing.

My father died in hospital because he needed to be there to make the whole process easier and because of his particular conditions.

We really had a great experience.

Myself and my sister held him as he passed.

We told him it was OK to go, his work was done and we were all around him.

That is what his soul wanted.

He was ready to go and we had the awareness to give him the space to express that.

His life had not been the easiest and he had struggled with it because he did not realise his own worth maybe.

As a consequence of that, we also struggled.

In the week before he died, there was healing for him and for us I think.

I realised that he had done the best that he knew how to do. If we criticise our parents as we go on the journey of awakening, we need to remember that they did the best they could for where they were at in their lives.

Other souls do not pass with an audience.

They slip away when there is no one around.

They choose that.

If you were not there, that is how it was meant to be.

I understand that people are disappointed if they "miss" that moment but if we can accept that the person themselves chooses that, that missed moment becomes easier to bear.

In any case, their energy can often still be felt even some time after that final breath has been taken.

Lots of people attest to that.

If you have a loved one near the end of this phase of existence, have the courage to assist them on their way.

Go with your own intuition.

Ask them what they want.

Do they really need to be moved to an unfamiliar environment?

Can what they need be administered in their own bed?

Can we take time out of our schedules to do this most valuable of work?

We are their voice at this most vulnerable of times.

They need us to step up.

We will be all the richer for the experience.

I know I am and there was great learning in it for me.

I hasten to add that this can be the case in a medical environment as well as long as we hold our own centre and ask for what we want.

We are the authority that speaks for our loved ones.

We should not surrender that unless absolutely necessary.

In some circumstances, we have to look on death from afar because we are not the next of kin, because of family trauma, relationship breakdowns, distance etc… We can really help the dying wo/man in that scenario as well with our thoughts and intentions.

That is the power of prayer.

We can be close to them in thought and love so we need to remember that.

We are always in the perfect place at the perfect time.

Isn't it great to know that?

When you were born, you cried and the world rejoiced. Live your life so that when you die the world cries and you rejoice – Native American Proverb

What have I Come to Know for Sure?

The short answer to the above is nothing!!!

However, I have come to a great realisation that with age does indeed come "wisdom" if we are brave enough to allow it in.

With age comes Ease.
With age comes Transformation.
With age comes Beauty.
With age comes Wealth.
With age comes Power.
With age comes Love.
With age comes Peace.
With age comes Joy.
With age comes Me.

What do I mean by all of this? I mean that aging is one of the greatest gifts that life can give us, in my opinion.

This belief helps me to find joy in everyday, peace with where I am in my life and the wonderful realisation that the more I age, the more these gifts increase.

Many people are denied the privilege of getting old as we all know very well.

How is it then that the world tells us the exact opposite about the aging process?

It is cloaked in the negative, seen as loss rather than gain and we are encouraged to disguise it at all costs.

This can be done with paint and powder, botox and even the scalpel.

This viewpoint is true of the Western World at least.

On the other hand, most of the native tribes and cultures around the globe have a different truth about aging.

Their elders are respected and even revered whereas we allow ours to disappear behind walls of dismissal.

Look at the faces of the elders around you in a new light. Take the time to sit with them and allow them the time to express what's in their hearts. Most of us are too busy with our own lives to really BE with them. We believe that they do not understand the modern world. We may be surprised by what they have to say.

Smart people learn from everything and everyone, average people from their experiences, stupid people already have all the answers – Socrates

A Final Word

We can begin to do things differently by critically observing our behaviour.

We can start by going behind our actions to see what is really driving them.

It's ultimately about taking responsibility for our own lives and the lives of those we love, who may not have the wherewithal to speak up for themselves.

You will probably need help to do a lot of this work.

Your friends will not be able to help you unless they have done training in these fields but often if they are too close to us, it does not work.

As I have already said, when you make the decision to do better, the teachers will show up in front of you.

Also as already stated, it is not for the faint-hearted.

We have been told and made to believe that we "are" faint-hearted but it is not true.

If we can begin to appreciate our amazing capabilities, profound changes can take place in our lives.

These may not be noticed by the outside world as many of them are internal.

I guarantee that your whole energy will change for the better and people will know that there is something different about you.

What will occur in any case is that you will care less and less about what other people think about you.

This will not be done in arrogance but in empowerment, compassion and good humour hopefully.

It is actually funny to see people's reactions when you change or refuse to be triggered like before.

I do it by jokingly saying things like "OK, tell me what to do with my life"!!!

However, more usually I just nod and smile when the unsolicited advice comes at me.

People's intentions, for the most part, are good.

Those intentions are often a reflection of the other person's fears and insecurities, and have very little to do with you.

That usually enables me to stay in open-heart mode and not get into the negativity of judgement and criticism.

I hasten to add that I am fully human and sometimes I do go back into old patterns.

That is OK too.

I am not yet perfect but rather perfect in my imperfection.

As I draw to the end of this most exciting project called "Book", I leave you with the hope that you will begin to find glimpses of your true self and bravely continue the journey of discovery.

Brava women!

Bravo men!

To know thyself is the beginning of wisdom – Socrates